The Silent Killer Diseases: Heart Disease, Cancer And Hypertension

Andrea Herrera

Table Of Contents

Chapter 1

Silent Killer Diseases

The silent executioner illness is a condition that has little to no side effects yet has the potential to be fatal if left untreated.

Major silent killer diseases include hypertension, cancer, and heart disease.

Other uncommon but serious disorders include essential amyloidosis, renal cell disease, pancreatic cancer, and infection with hepatitis B or C, to name a few.

The biggest silent killer disease is coronary diseases. The main risk factors increase risks like elevated cholesterol.

For silent killer diseases including malignant growths and cardiac ailment, smoking is a major risk factor. In the lungs, 87% of cellular breakdowns are a result of smoking.

Heart Ailments

Why Do Heart Infections Occur?

Any ailment affecting the heart or cardiovascular system is referred to as a coronary illness.
There are several types, some of which are preventable.

Kinds Of Heart Infections

There are a few unique sorts of coronary illnesses, and they influence the heart and veins in various ways.

The segments beneath check out a few distinct sorts of coronary illness in more detail.

Coronary corridor illness

Coronary corridor illness, otherwise called coronary illness, is the most widely recognized kind of coronary illness.

It is created when the courses that supply blood to the heart become obstructed with plaque. This makes them solidify and limit. Plaque contains cholesterol and different substances.

Subsequently, the blood supply diminishes, and the heart gets less oxygen and fewer supplements. In time, the heart muscle debilitates, and there is a gamble of cardiovascular breakdown and arrhythmias.

At the point when plaque develops in the courses, it is called atherosclerosis. Plaque in the supply routes can burst from blockages and cause the bloodstream to stop, which can prompt coronary failure.

Inborn Heart Disease

An individual with an inborn heart deformity is brought into the world with a heart issue. There are many sorts of intrinsic heart abandons which include:

Abnormal heart valves: Valves may not open as expected, or they might spill blood.

Septal imperfections: There is an opening in the wall between either the lower chambers or the upper offices of the heart.

Atresia: One of the heart valves is absent.
Intrinsic coronary illness can include major underlying issues, like the shortfall of a ventricle or issues with surprising associations between the primary courses that leave the heart.

Numerous intrinsic heart surrenders cause no perceptible side effects and just become evident during a standard clinical check.

As per the American Heart Affiliation (AHA), heart mumbles frequently influence kids, however, just because of a deformity.

Arrhythmia
Arrhythmia alludes to a sporadic heartbeat. It happens when the electrical motivations that coordinate the heartbeat don't work accurately. Thus, the heart might thump excessively fast, too leisurely, or unpredictably.

There are different kinds of arrhythmias, including:

Tachycardia: This alludes to a fast heartbeat.
Bradycardia: This alludes to a sluggish heartbeat.
Untimely withdrawals: This alludes to an early heartbeat.
Atrial fibrillation: This is a kind of unpredictable heartbeat.
An individual might see an inclination like a rippling or a dashing heart.

At times, arrhythmias can be dangerous or have extreme confusion.

Widened cardiomyopathy

In widened cardiomyopathy, the heart chambers become enlarged, implying that the heart muscle extends and becomes more slender. The most widely recognized reasons for widened cardiomyopathy are past respiratory failures, arrhythmias, and poisons, however, hereditary qualities can likewise assume a part.

Accordingly, the heart becomes more fragile and can't siphon blood as expected. It can bring about arrhythmia, blood clumps in the heart, and cardiovascular breakdown.
It typically influences individuals who matured 20-60 years.

Myocardial dead tissue
Otherwise called coronary failure, myocardial dead tissue includes an interference of the bloodstream to the heart. This can harm or annihilate some portion of the heart muscle.

The most well-known reason for respiratory failure is plaque, blood coagulation, or both in a coronary course. It can likewise happen on the off chance that a vein unexpectedly limits or fits.

Cardiovascular breakdown
At the point when an individual has a cardiovascular breakdown, their heart is as yet

working, yet not as well as it ought to be. The congestive cardiovascular breakdown is a sort of cardiovascular breakdown that can happen from issues with the siphoning or loosening up capability.

A cardiovascular breakdown can result from untreated coronary conduit illness, hypertension, arrhythmias, and different circumstances. These circumstances can influence the heart's capacity to siphon or unwind appropriately.

Cardiovascular breakdown can be hazardous, yet looking for early treatment for heart-related conditions can assist with forestalling inconveniences.

Hypertrophic cardiomyopathy

This condition as a rule creates when a hereditary issue influences the heart muscle. It will in general be an acquired condition.

The walls of the muscle thicken, and withdrawals become more diligently. This influences the heart's capacity to take in and siphon out blood. At times, a check can happen.

There might be no side effects, and many individuals don't get a finding. Nonetheless, hypertrophic cardiomyopathy can deteriorate over the long haul and lead to different heart issues.

Anybody with a family background of this condition ought to request a screening, as getting treatment can assist with forestalling confusion.

Hypertrophic cardiomyopathy is the primary driver of heart demise among youngsters and competitors under 35 years of age, as indicated by the AHA.

Mitral valve spewing forth

This occasion happens when the mitral valve in the heart doesn't close firmly enough and permits blood to stream once again into the heart.

Thus, blood can't travel through the heart or body productively, and it can come down to the offices of the heart. In time, the heart can become developed, and cardiovascular breakdown can result

Mitral valve prolapse

This happens when the valve folds of the mitral valve don't close as expected. All things being equal, they swell into the left chamber. This can cause a heart to mumble.

Mitral valve prolapse isn't typically perilous, however, certain individuals might have to get treatment for it.

Hereditary elements and connective tissue issues can cause this condition, which influences around 2% of the populace.

Aortic stenosis

In aortic stenosis, the aspiratory valve is thick or combined and doesn't open accurately. This makes it difficult for the heart to siphon blood from the left ventricle into the aorta.

An individual might be brought into the world with it because of inherent inconsistencies of the valve, or it might foster after some time because of calcium stores or scarring.

Side Effects Of Heart Infections

The side effects of coronary illness rely upon the particular sort an individual has. Additionally, some heart conditions cause no side effects by any means.

A few signs and side effects that could demonstrate coronary episode include:

Side effects

Coronary illness side effects rely upon the kind of coronary illness.

In youngsters, the side effects of an inborn heart imperfection might incorporate cyanosis, a blue hint to the skin, and a failure to work out.

Side effects Of Heart Sicknesses In The Veins

Coronary course illness is a typical heart condition that influences the significant veins that supply the heart muscle.

Cholesterol stores (plaques) in the heart courses are generally the reason for coronary vein sickness. The development of these plaques is called atherosclerosis.

Atherosclerosis lessens the bloodstream to the heart and different pieces of the body. It can prompt a coronary episode, chest torment (angina), or stroke.

Coronary vein infection side effects might be different for people. For example, men are bound to have chest torment. Ladies are bound to have different side effects alongside chest uneasiness, like windedness, sickness, and outrageous weakness.

Side effects of coronary supply route sickness can include:

Chest torment, chest snugness, chest tension, and chest uneasiness (angina)

Windedness
Undeniable annoyance, jaw, throat, upper gut region, or back
Torment, deadness, shortcoming, or chilliness in the legs or arms assuming the veins in those body regions are limited
You probably won't be determined to have coronary corridor infection until you have a coronary failure, angina, stroke, or cardiovascular breakdown. It's vital to look for heart side effects and talk about worries with your medical care supplier. Heart (cardiovascular) illness can in some cases be seen as ahead of schedule with standard wellbeing tests.

Respiratory failure can prompt heart failure, which is the point at which the heart stops and the body can never again work. Individual require quick clinical consideration if they have any side effects of a respiratory failure.

Causes And Chance Elements

Coronary illness creates when there is:

Harm to all or part of the heart
an issue with the veins prompting or from the heart
A low stockpile of oxygen and supplements for the heart
An issue with the mood of the heart
At times, there is a hereditary reason.
Be that as it may, some way of life variables and ailments can likewise build the gamble. These include:
Hypertension
Elevated cholesterol
Smoking
A high admission of liquor
Overweight and corpulence
Diabetes
Family background of coronary illness
Dietary decisions
Age
A past filled with toxemia during pregnancy
Low action levels
Rest apnea
High pressure and uneasiness levels

Defective heart valves

The World Wellbeing Association (WHO) specifies neediness and stress as two key variables adding to a worldwide expansion in heart and cardiovascular illness.

Medication

The treatment choices will differ contingent upon the sort of coronary illness an individual has, however, a few normal methodologies incorporate making way of life changes, taking meds, and going through a medical procedure.

Prescriptions

Different prescriptions can assist with treating heart conditions. The principal choices include:

Anticoagulants: Otherwise called blood thinners, these prescriptions can forestall clusters. They incorporate warfarin (Coumadin) and the immediate oral anticoagulants dabigatran, rivaroxaban, and apixaban.

Antiplatelet treatments: These incorporate anti-inflammatory medicine, and they can likewise forestall clumps.

Angiotensin-changing over compound inhibitors: These can assist with treating cardiovascular breakdown and hypertension by making the veins extend. Lisinopril is one model.

Angiotensin II receptor blockers: These can likewise control circulatory strain. Losartan is one model.
Angiotensin receptor neprilysin inhibitors: These can assist with emptying the heart and intrude on the compound pathways that debilitate it.

Beta-blockers: Metoprolol and different drugs in this class can diminish the pulse and lower circulatory strain. They can likewise treat arrhythmias and angina.

Calcium channel blockers: These can bring down circulatory strain and forestall arrhythmias by decreasing the siphoning strength of the heart and loosening up the veins. One model is diltiazem (Cardizem).

Cholesterol-bringing down prescriptions: Statins, like atorvastatin (Lipitor), and different sorts of medications can assist with decreasing degrees of low-thickness lipoprotein cholesterol in the body.

Digitalis: Arrangements like digoxin (Lanoxin) can build the strength of the heart's siphoning activity. They can likewise assist with treating cardiovascular breakdown and arrhythmias.

Diuretics: These drugs can diminish the heart's responsibility, lower circulatory strain, and eliminate the abundance of water from the body. Furosemide (Lasix) is one model.

Vasodilators: These are meds to bring down circulatory strain. They do this by loosening up the veins. Dynamite (Nitrostat) is one model. These meds can likewise assist with facilitating

chest torment. Become familiar with vasodilation here.
A specialist will work with the person to track down a reasonable choice.

Now and then, incidental effects happen. If so, assessing the medicine regimen might be important.

Medical procedure
Going through a heart medical procedure can assist with treating blockages and heart issues when drugs are not viable.

A few normal kinds of the medical procedure include:

Coronary course sidesteps a medical procedure: This permits the bloodstream to arrive at a piece of the heart when a supply route is impeded.
Coronary supply route sidesteps joining is the most widely recognized medical procedure. A specialist can utilize a solid vein from one more piece of the body to fix an impeded one.

Coronary angiography: This is a strategy that extends restricted or hindered coronary veins. It is frequently joined with the inclusion of a stent, which is a wire-network tube that permits a more straightforward bloodstream.

Valve substitution or fix: A specialist can supplant or fix a valve that isn't working accurately.

Fix a medical procedure: A specialist can fix inborn heart imperfections, aneurysms, and different issues.
Gadget implantation: Pacemakers, swell catheters, and different gadgets can assist with directing the heartbeat and backing the bloodstream.

Laser treatment: Transmyocardial laser revascularization can assist with treating angina.
Labyrinth medical procedure: A specialist can make new ways for electrical signs to go

through. This can assist with treating atrial fibrillation.

Anticipation

Some way of life measures can assist with diminishing the gamble of coronary illness. These include:

Eating a reasonable eating regimen: Pick a heart-sound eating routine that is wealthy in fiber and favors entire grains and new foods grown from the ground. The Mediterranean eating regimen and the Scramble diet might be great for heart wellbeing. Likewise, it might assist with restricting the admission of handled food sources and added fat, salt, and sugar.

Practicing consistently: This can assist with fortifying the heart and circulatory framework, lessen cholesterol, and keep up with the pulse.

Stopping or abstaining from smoking: Smoking is a significant gamble factor for heart and cardiovascular circumstances.

Restricting liquor consumption: Ladies ought to polish off something like one standard beverage each day, and men ought to polish off something like two standard beverages each day.

Overseeing fundamental circumstances: Look for treatment for conditions that influence heart wellbeing, for example, hypertension, heftiness, and diabetes.

Making these strides can assist with helping generally speaking well-being and diminish the gamble of coronary illness and its complexities.

Standpoint

Coronary illness is a typical medical condition.

There are a few unique sorts of coronary illnesses. Some come from hereditary issues and are not preventable.

Much of the time, nonetheless, an individual can do whatever it takes to forestall coronary illness and its intricacies. These means incorporate following a solid eating regimen, getting a lot of activity, and looking for exhortation when the principal side effects of coronary illness show up.

Chapter 2

Cancer Disease

The Definition of Cancer

Malignant growth is a sickness wherein a portion of the body's cells develop wildly and spread to different pieces of the body.

Malignant growth can begin anyplace in the human body, which is comprised of trillions of cells. Ordinarily, human cells develop and duplicate (through a cycle called cell division) to shape new cells as the body needs them. At the point when cells become old or become harmed, they pass on, and new cells have their spot.

Once in a while, this precise cycle separates, and strange or harmed cells develop and duplicate when they shouldn't. These cells might shape growths, which are pieces of tissue. Growths can be dangerous or not destructive (harmless).

Harmful growths spread into, or attack, close by tissues and can venture out to far-off places in the body to shape new growths (a cycle called metastasis). Carcinogenic cancers may likewise be called dangerous growths. Numerous malignant growths structure strong growths, however diseases of the blood, like leukemias, for the most part, don't.

Harmless cancers don't spread into, or attack, close by tissues. At the point when eliminated, harmless cancers normally don't bounce back, though malignant growths in some cases do. Harmless growths can here and there be very huge, in any case. Some can cause serious side effects or be perilous, like harmless growths in the mind.

Contrasts Between Disease Cells And Typical Cells

Malignant growth cells vary from ordinary cells in numerous ways.

For example, malignant growth cells:

Fill without any signs advising them to develop.

Typical cells possibly develop when they get such signals.
Ordinary cells quit developing when they experience different cells, and most typical cells don't move around the body.
These veins supply growths with oxygen and supplements and eliminate side effects from cancers.
The insusceptible framework regularly dispenses with harmed or strange cells.
Stunt the insusceptible framework into assisting disease cells with remaining alive and developing.

For example, some malignant growth cells persuade safe cells to safeguard cancer as opposed to going after it.
What's more, some malignant growth cells make energy from supplements in another way than most typical cells. This lets disease cells develop all the more rapidly.
Commonly, malignant growth cells depend so vigorously on these strange ways of behaving that they can't make do without them.

For instance, some disease treatments keep veins from developing toward growth, basically keeping cancer from required supplements.

How Does Malignant growth Create?

Malignant growth is made by specific changes in qualities, the fundamental actual units of legacy. Qualities are organized in lengthy strands of firmly stuffed DNA called chromosomes.

Malignant growth is a hereditary illness — that is, it is brought about by changes to qualities that control how our cell's capability, particularly how they develop and partition.

Hereditary changes that cause disease can happen because:

Of blunders that happen as cells partition.

Of harm to DNA brought about by hurtful substances in the climate, for example, the synthetics in tobacco smoke and bright beams from the sun. (Our Malignant growth Causes and Anticipation area has more data.)

They were acquired from our folks.

The body regularly wipes out cells with harmed DNA before they turn malignant. Yet, the body's capacity to do so goes down as we age. This is important for the motivation behind why there is a higher endanger of disease further down the road.

Every individual's malignant growth has a special mix of hereditary changes. As the disease keeps on developing, extra changes will happen. Indeed, even inside similar cancer, various cells might have different hereditary changes.

Sorts Of Qualities That Cause Disease

The hereditary changes that add to malignant growth will generally influence three fundamental kinds of qualities — proto-oncogenes, cancer silencer qualities, and DNA-fix qualities. These progressions are now and again called "drivers" of disease.

Proto-oncogenes are associated with ordinary cell development and division. Nonetheless, when these qualities are adjusted in some ways or are more dynamic than typical, they might become disease-causing qualities (or oncogenes), permitting cells to develop and endure when they shouldn't.

Cancer silencer qualities are additionally engaged with controlling cell development and division. Cells with specific changes in cancer silencer qualities might separate in an uncontrolled way.

DNA fix qualities are engaged with fixing harmed DNA. Cells with transformations in these qualities will generally foster extra changes in different qualities and changes in their chromosomes, for example, duplications and cancellations of chromosome parts. Together, these changes might make the cells harmful.

As researchers have more deeply studied the sub-atomic changes that lead to malignant growth, they have found that specific transformations regularly happen in many kinds of diseases. Presently there are numerous disease therapies accessible that target quality transformations tracked down in malignant growth. A couple of these therapies can be utilized by anybody with a disease that has the designated transformation, regardless of where the malignant growth began developing.

In metastasis, disease cells split away from where they first shaped and structure new cancers in quite a while of the body.
A malignant growth that has spread from where it was previously framed to somewhere else in the body is called metastatic disease. The interaction by which disease cells spread to different pieces of the body is called metastasis.

Metastatic disease has a similar name and similar kind of malignant growth cells as the first, or essential, disease. For instance, a bosom disease that frames a metastatic growth in the lung is metastatic, not cellular breakdown in the lungs.

Under a magnifying lens, metastatic disease cells for the most part look equivalent to cells of the first malignant growth. In addition, metastatic disease cells and cells of the first malignant growth normally share a few sub-atomic elements practically speaking, for example, the presence of explicit chromosome changes.

At times, therapy might assist with dragging out the existence of individuals with metastatic disease. In different cases, the essential objective of therapy for metastatic disease is to control the development of malignant growth or to alleviate the side effects it is causing. Metastatic growths can make serious harm how the body's capabilities and the vast majority who pass on from malignant growth pass on from metastatic illness.

Tissue Changes that Are Not Disease

Only one out of every odd change in the body's tissues is a disease. Some tissue changes might form into malignant growth if they are not treated, nonetheless. Here are a few instances of tissue changes that are not malignant growth but rather, at times, are observed because they could become disease:

Hyperplasia happens when cells inside a tissue duplicate quicker than typical and additional cells develop. In any case, the cells and how the tissue is coordinated still look ordinary under a magnifying lens. Hyperplasia can be brought about by a few factors or conditions, including constant bothering.

Dysplasia is a further developed condition than hyperplasia. In dysplasia, there is likewise a development of additional cells. In any case, the cells look unusual and there are changes in how the tissue is coordinated. As a rule, the more unusual the cells and tissue look, the more prominent the opportunity that disease will shape. A few sorts of dysplasia might be checked or treated, yet others don't. An

illustration of dysplasia is an unusual mole (called a dysplastic nevus) that structures on the skin. A dysplastic nevus can transform into melanoma, albeit most don't.
Carcinoma in situ is a much further developed condition. Although it is once in a while called stage 0 malignant growth, it isn't a disease because the strange cells don't attack close by tissue the way that disease cells do. But since certain carcinomas in situ may become a disease, they are generally treated.

Ordinary cells might become malignant growth cells. Before malignant growth cells structure in tissues of the body, the phones go through unusual changes called hyperplasia and dysplasia. In hyperplasia, there is an expansion in the number of cells in an organ or tissue that seem typical under a magnifying lens. In dysplasia, the cells look unusual under a magnifying lens however are not a disease. Hyperplasia and dysplasia could become diseases.

Kinds Of Malignant Growth

There are over 100 kinds of malignant growth. Kinds of a malignant growth are typically named for the organs or tissues where the diseases is structure. For instance, cellular breakdown in the lungs begins in the lung, and mind disease begins in the cerebrum. Diseases likewise might be portrayed by the sort of cell that shaped them, like an epithelial cell or a squamous cell.

Here are a few classifications of diseases that start in unambiguous sorts of cells:

Carcinoma

Carcinomas are the most well-known sort of malignant growth. They are shaped by epithelial cells, which are the cells that cover within and outside surfaces of the body. There are many sorts of epithelial cells, which frequently have a segment-like shape when seen under a magnifying lens.

Carcinomas that start in various epithelial cell types have explicit names:

Adenocarcinoma is a disease that structures in epithelial cells that produce liquids or bodily fluid. Tissues with this sort of epithelial cell are some of the time called glandular tissues. Most diseases of the bosom, colon, and prostate are adenocarcinomas.

Basal cell carcinoma is a disease that starts in the lower or basal (base) layer of the epidermis, which is an individual's external layer of skin.

Squamous cell carcinoma is a malignant growth that structures in squamous cells, which are epithelial cells that lie just underneath the external surface of the skin. Squamous cells likewise line numerous different organs, including the stomach, digestion tracts, lungs, bladder, and kidneys. Squamous cells look level, similar to fish scales when seen under a magnifying instrument. Squamous cell carcinomas are at times called epidermoid carcinomas.

Momentary cell carcinoma is a malignant growth that structures in a kind of epithelial tissue called the temporary epithelium or urothelium. This tissue, which is comprised of many layers of epithelial cells that can get greater and more modest, is tracked down in the linings of the bladder, ureters, part of the kidneys (renal pelvis), and a couple of different organs. A few tumors of the bladder, ureters, and kidneys are temporary cell carcinomas.

Osteosarcoma is the most well-known disease of bone. The most widely recognized sorts of delicate tissue sarcoma are leiomyosarcoma, Kaposi sarcoma, threatening sinewy histiocytoma, liposarcoma, and dermatofibrosarcoma protuberans.

Leukemia

Tumors that start in the blood-shaping tissue of the bone marrow are called leukemias. These malignant growths don't frame strong cancers. All things considered, huge quantities of strange white platelets (leukemia cells and leukemic impact cells) develop in the blood and bone marrow, swarming out ordinary platelets. The low degree of typical platelets can make it harder for the body to get oxygen to its tissues, control dying, or battle diseases.

There are four normal sorts of leukemia, which are assembled in light of how rapidly the illness deteriorates (intense or persistent) and on the kind of platelet, the malignant growth begins in (lymphoblastic or myeloid). Intense types of leukemia develop rapidly and persistent structures develop all the more leisurely.

Lymphoma

Lymphoma is a malignant growth that starts in lymphocytes (Immune system microorganisms or B cells). These are infection-battling white platelets that are essential for the invulnerable framework. In lymphoma, unusual lymphocytes develop in lymph hubs and lymph vessels, as well as in different organs of the body.

There are two principal sorts of lymphoma:

Hodgkin lymphoma - Individuals with this sickness have unusual lymphocytes that are called Reed-Sternberg cells. These cells for the most part structure from B cells.

Non-Hodgkin lymphoma - This is a huge gathering of tumors that begin in lymphocytes. The diseases can develop rapidly or gradually and can frame from B cells or Lymphocytes.

Numerous Myeloma

Numerous myeloma is a malignant growth that starts in plasma cells, one more kind of resistant cell. The unusual plasma cells, called myeloma cells, develop in the bone marrow and structure cancers in bones generally through the body. Different myeloma is likewise called plasma cell myeloma and Kahler sickness.

Melanoma

Melanoma is a disease that starts in cells that become melanocytes, which are particular cells that make melanin (the shade that gives skin its tone). Most melanomas structure on the skin, yet melanomas can likewise frame in other pigmented tissues, like the eye.

Cerebrum and Spinal String Growths

There are various kinds of mind and spinal rope growths. These cancers are named in light of the kind of cell in which they are shaped and where the growth is originally framed in the focal sensory system. For instance, astrocytic cancer starts in star-molded synapses called astrocytes, which assist with keeping nerve cells solid. Cerebrum growths can be harmless (not disease) or dangerous (disease).

Different Sorts of Cancers

Microbe Cell Cancers

Microbe cell cancers are a kind of growth that starts in the cells that lead to sperm or eggs. These growths can happen anyplace in the body and can be either harmless or dangerous.

Neuroendocrine Cancers

Neuroendocrine cancers structure from cells that discharge chemicals into the blood in light of a sign from the sensory system. These growths, which might make higher-than-typical measures of chemicals, can cause a wide range of side effects. Neuroendocrine cancers might be harmless or threatening.

Carcinoid Cancers

Carcinoid cancers are a kind of neuroendocrine growth. They are slow-developing cancers that are generally tracked down in the gastrointestinal framework (most frequently in the rectum and small digestive system). Carcinoid growths might spread to the liver or different locales in the body, and they might emit substances like serotonin or prostaglandins, causing carcinoid conditions.

Side effects

Signs and side effects brought about by malignant growth will fluctuate contingent upon which piece of the body is impacted.

A few general signs and side effects related to, however not well defined for, disease, include:

Exhaustion

Bump or area of thickening that can be felt under the skin

Weight changes, including accidental misfortune or gain

Skin changes, for example, yellowing, obscuring or redness of the skin, bruises that will not recuperate, or changes to existing moles

Changes in entrail or bladder propensities

Persevering hack or inconvenience relaxing

Trouble gulping

Dryness

Tireless heartburn or inconvenience after eating

Tireless, unexplained muscle or joint torment

Constant, unexplained fevers or night sweats

Unexplained draining or swelling

When to see a specialist

Make a meeting with your primary care physician assuming you have any industrious signs or side effects that worry you.

On the off chance that you have no signs or side effects, but are stressed over your gamble of disease, examine your interests with your primary care physician. Get some information about which disease screening tests and systems are proper for you.

Causes

Malignant growth is brought about by changes (transformations) to the DNA inside cells. The DNA inside a cell is bundled into countless individual qualities, every one of which contains a bunch of directions advising the cell which capabilities to perform, as well as how to develop and partition. Mistakes in the guidelines can make the cell stop its not unexpected capability and may permit a cell to become destructive.

What do quality changes do?

A quality transformation can educate a sound cell to:

Permit fast development. A quality transformation can advise a cell to develop and partition all the more quickly. This makes numerous new cells that all have that equivalent transformation.

Neglect to stop uncontrolled cell development. Ordinary cells know when to quit developing so you have the perfect number of each kind of cell. Disease cells lose the controls (cancer silencer qualities) that let them know when to quit developing. A transformation in a growth silencer quality permits disease cells to keep developing and gathering.

Commit errors while fixing DNA blunders. DNA fix qualities search for blunders in a cell's DNA and make remedies. A change in a DNA fix quality might imply that different blunders aren't revised, driving cells to become harmful.

These transformations are the most widely recognized ones tracked down in malignant growth. Be that as it may, numerous other quality transformations can add to causing disease.

What causes quality changes?

Quality transformations can happen in light of multiple factors, for example:

Quality changes you're brought into the world with. You might be brought into the world with a hereditary change that you acquired from your folks. This sort of transformation represents a little level of malignant growth.

Quality changes that happen after birth. Most quality changes happen after you're conceived and aren't acquired. Various powers can cause quality changes, like smoking, radiation, infections, malignant growth causing synthetics (cancer-causing agents), heftiness, chemicals, persistent irritation, and an absence of activity.

Risk factors

While specialists have thought of what might build your gamble of malignant growth, most diseases happen in individuals who have no realized gambling factors. Factors known to build your gamble of malignant growth include:

Your age

The disease can require a long time to create. That is the reason a great many people determined to have malignant growth are 65 or more established. While it's more considered normal in more seasoned grown-ups, malignant growth isn't only a grown-up illness — the disease can be analyzed at whatever stage in life.

Your propensities

A certain way of life decision is known to expand your gamble of disease. Smoking, drinking more than one beverage daily for ladies and up to two beverages per day for men, unnecessary openness to the sun or continuous rankling sun-related burns, being fat, and having hazardous sex can add to disease.

You can address these propensities to bring down your gamble of disease — however, a few propensities are more straightforward to change than others.

Your family ancestry

Just a little part of malignant growths are because of an acquired condition. Assuming disease is normal in your family, it's conceivable that changes are being passed starting with one age and then onto the next. You may be a possibility so that hereditary testing could see whether you have acquired changes that could build your gamble of specific malignant growths. Remember that having an acquired hereditary change doesn't be guaranteed to mean you'll get malignant growth.

Your medical issue

Some persistent medical issues, like ulcerative colitis, can notably build your gamble of fostering specific tumors. Converse with your PCP about your gamble.

Your current circumstance

The climate around you might contain destructive synthetic compounds that can expand your gamble of disease. Regardless of whether you smoke, you could breathe in handed-down cigarette smoke assuming that you go where individuals are smoking or on the other hand on the off chance that you live with somebody who smokes. Synthetic compounds in your home or working environment, like asbestos and benzene, additionally are related to an expanded gamble of disease.

Inconveniences

Disease and its treatment can cause a few intricacies, including:

Torment. Torment can be brought about by malignant growth or by disease therapy, however not all disease is excruciating. Drugs and different methodologies can treat disease-related torment.

Weariness. Weariness in individuals with malignant growth has many causes, yet it can frequently be made due. Weariness related to chemotherapy or radiation treatment therapies is normal, yet all at once, it's typically brief.

Trouble relaxing. Disease or malignant growth treatment might cause a sensation of being winded. Medicines might bring help.

Queasiness. Certain malignant growths and disease medicines can cause sickness. Your PCP can now and again anticipate on the off chance that your treatment is probably going to cause queasiness. Meds and different medicines might help you forestall or diminish queasiness.

Loose bowels or clogging. Disease and malignant growth treatment can influence your entrails and cause looseness of the bowels or blockage.

Weight reduction. Disease and malignant growth treatment might cause weight reduction. The disease takes food from typical cells and denies them supplements. This is frequently not impacted by the number of calories or what sort of food is eaten; it's hard to treat. Much of the time, utilizing counterfeit nourishment through tubes into the stomach or vein doesn't assist with changing weight reduction.

Compound changes in your body: Disease can agitate the typical substance balance in your body and increment your gamble of serious confusion. Signs and side effects of compound lopsided characteristics could incorporate extreme thirst, continuous pee, obstruction, and disarray.

Mind and sensory system issues: Disease can push on adjacent nerves and cause agony and loss of capability of one piece of your body. Malignant growth that includes the mind can cause cerebral pains and stroke-like signs and side effects, like shortcomings on one side of your body.

Uncommon safe framework responses to disease: at times the body's invulnerable framework might respond to the presence of malignant growth by going after solid cells. Called paraneoplastic disorders, these exceptionally intriguing responses can prompt various signs and side effects, for example, trouble strolling and seizures.

Malignant growth that spreads: As the disease progresses, it might spread (metastasize) to different pieces of the body. Where malignant growth spreads relies upon the kind of disease.

Malignant growth that profits: Disease survivors have a gamble of malignant growth repeat. A few tumors are bound to repeat more than others. Get some information about how you might decrease your gamble of malignant growth repeat. Your PCP might devise a subsequent consideration plan for you after treatment. This plan might remember occasional sweeps and tests for the long periods after your therapy, to search for malignant growth repeat.

Counteraction

Specialists have distinguished multiple ways of decreasing your gamble of disease, for example,

Quit smoking. Assuming that you smoke, quit. If you don't smoke, don't begin. Smoking is connected to a few kinds of disease — not simply a cellular breakdown in the lungs. Halting now will diminish your gamble of disease later on.
Keep away from inordinate sun openness. Hurtful bright ultra Violet beams from the sun can expand your gamble of skin malignant growth. Limit your sun openness by remaining in the shade, wearing defensive attire, or applying sunscreen.

Eat a solid eating routine: Pick an eating routine wealthy in foods grown from the ground. Select entire grains and lean proteins. Limit your admission of handled meats.
Practice most days of the week. Ordinary activity is connected to a lower hazard of malignant growth. If you haven't been practicing routinely, begin gradually and move gradually for as long as 30 minutes or longer.

Keep a solid weight: Being overweight or hefty may build your gamble of malignant growth. Work to accomplish and keep a sound load through a mix of a solid eating routine and normal activity.

Savor liquor balance: assuming you decide to drink. If you decide to drink liquor, do as such with some restraint. For sound grown-ups, that implies depending upon one beverage daily for ladies and up to two beverages per day for men.

Plan disease screening tests. Converse with your doctor, about what sorts of disease screening tests are best for you in light of your gamble factors.

Get some information about vaccinations. Certain infections increment your gamble of malignant growth. Inoculations might assist with forestalling those infections, including hepatitis B, which expands the gamble of liver malignant growth, and human papillomavirus (HPV), which builds the gamble of cervical disease and different tumors. Find out if inoculation against these infections is fitting for you.

Is There A Remedy For Malignant growth?

At the point when you have the disease or care about somebody who does, "fix" might be the word you need to hear more than some other. It's likewise a word most specialists won't say.

Dissimilar to different sicknesses, malignant growth has its language: There's no remedy for it, yet there are therapies that might have the option to fix certain individuals of certain tumors.

At the point when you comprehend the distinction, it has a significant effect.

"Natural product" is a general term you use to cover a wide range of sorts: apples, cranberries, pineapple and that's just the beginning.

Similarly, "malignant growth" is a trick all words for over 200 sorts, including tumors of the bladder, cerebrum, bosom, colon, eye, kidney, liver, lungs, ovaries, and skin.

At the point when you have the disease, unusual cells create, partition, and obliterate solid tissue in your body. A few kinds develop gradually; others spread rapidly. Every caring begins in an alternate piece of your body and has its grades, stages, and side effects.

Since each sort of malignant growth is unique, there's no one-size-fits-all fix. However, some of the time, individuals might say they are restored assuming that their malignant growth appears to disappear with treatment. In any case, it's not exactly that straightforward.

Chapter 3

Hypertension

The heart is a muscle that siphons blood around the body. As it voyages, the blood conveys oxygen to the body's fundamental organs.

In some cases, an issue in the body makes it harder for the heart to siphon blood. For instance, this could happen if a conduit turns out to be excessively limited.

Persevering hypertension can overburden the walls of the corridors. This can prompt different medical conditions, some of which can life undermine.

Signs And Side effects

The vast majority with hypertension won't encounter any side effects, which is the reason individuals frequently consider hypertension the "quiet executioner."

Be that as it may, when pulse comes to around 180/120 mm Hg, it turns into a hypertensive emergency, which is a health-related crisis.

At this stage, an individual might have:
Migraine
Queasiness
Spewing
Wooziness
Obscured or twofold vision
Nosebleeds
Heart palpitations
Shortness of breath
Anyone who encounters these side effects ought to look for sure-fire clinical consideration.

Side effects In Females
Hormonal elements imply that the gamble of hypertension might be different in guys and females.

Factors that can expand the gamble of hypertension in females include:
Pregnancy

Menopause
Utilizing conception prevention pills

During pregnancy, hypertension can demonstrate toxemia, a possibly perilous condition that can influence both the individual and their embryo.

Side effects of toxemia include:

Migraines
Vision changes
Stomach torment
Enlarging because of edema

Side effects In Teenagers And Individuals In Their Mid 20s
Teens can foster hypertension because of stoutness or a fundamental ailment.

Conceivable clinical variables include:
Parts of metabolic circumstances, like sort 2 diabetes
Kidney illness.
Endocrine illness influences the chemicals.

Vascular illness influences the veins.
A neurological condition.

Side effects in kids
Hypertension can influence kids. Having heftiness and diabetes expands the gamble, however other fundamental causes include:
Cancer.
Heart issues.
Kidney issues.
Obstructive rest apnea.
Rheumatologic jumble.
Thyroid issues.
A hereditary condition, like Cushing's disorder
Utilization of specific medications
Diet high in fat and salt.

Similarly, as with grown-ups, hypertension doesn't frequently cause side effects in kids.
Notwithstanding, assuming they happen, they might include:
Cerebral pain
Weariness
Mental changes or changes in mental status

Regurgitating

These side effects are probably going to demonstrate extreme hypertension.

They may likewise have indications of another condition.

Side effects in children
Infants and exceptionally youthful children can now and then have hypertension because of a fundamental medical issue, like kidney or coronary illness.

Any side effects might be vague or not observable, or hypertension might happen close by side effects of different circumstances.

A baby with hypertension may likewise insight:
Seizures
Crabbiness
Laziness
Taking care of issues
Fast relaxing

Apnea
Different side effects will rely upon the condition causing hypertension.

Reasons For Hypertension

Hypertension can happen when certain progressions occur in the body or on the other hand assuming an individual is brought into the world with explicit hereditary elements that cause a medical issue.

It can influence individuals with:
Stoutness
Type 2 diabetes
Kidney infection
Obstructive rest apnea
Lupus
Scleroderma
Underactive or overactive thyroid
Innate circumstances, like Cushing's disorder, acromegaly, or pheochromocytoma
In some cases, there is no clear reason. For this situation, a specialist will analyze essential hypertension.

Polishing off a low-fat eating regimen, keeping a moderate weight, lessening liquor utilization, and halting smoking tobacco, will assist with bringing down the gamble of hypertension.

Assuming you have hypertension, you might contemplate whether the drug is important to cut the numbers down. However, the way of life assumes a fundamental part in treating hypertension. Controlling circulatory strain with a solid way of life could forestall, delay or lessen the requirement for the drug.

Cure

The following are 10 way of life changes that can bring down the pulse and hold it down.

1. Lose additional pounds and watch your waistline

Pulse frequently increments as weight increments. Being overweight additionally can cause disturbed breathing while you rest (rest apnea), which further raises your pulse.

Weight reduction is one of the best ways of life changes for controlling pulse. On the off chance that you're overweight or have heftiness, losing even a limited quantity of weight can assist with a diminishing pulse. Additionally, the size of the waistline is significant. Conveying a lot of weight around the midriff can expand the gamble of hypertension.

2. Work-out consistently

Standard actual work can bring down hypertension. It's essential to continue to exercise to keep circulatory strain from rising once more.

Exercise can likewise assist with keeping raised circulatory strain from transforming into hypertension (hypertension). For people who have hypertension, normal active work can bring circulatory strain down to more secure levels.

A few instances of vigorous activity that can assist with bringing down pulse incorporate strolling, running, cycling, swimming, or moving. Another chance is to stop and do aerobic exercise. This kind of preparation includes rotating short eruptions of extraordinary action with times of lighter movement.

Strength preparation additionally can assist with decreasing circulatory strain. Plan to incorporate strength-preparing practices no less than two days every week. Converse with a medical care supplier about fostering an activity program.

3. Eat a solid eating routine

Eating an eating regimen wealthy in entire grains, natural products, vegetables, and low-fat dairy items and low in immersed fat and cholesterol can bring down hypertension. Instances of eating plans that can assist with controlling circulatory strain are the Dietary Ways to deal with Stop Hypertension (Run) diet and the Mediterranean eating routine.

4. Decrease salt (sodium) in your eating regimen

Indeed, even a little decrease of sodium in the eating routine can further develop heart well-being and lessen hypertension.
The impact of sodium consumption on circulatory strain shifts among gatherings.

To decrease sodium in the eating routine:
Peruse food marks. Search for low-sodium variants of food sources and drinks.
Eat less handled food varieties. Just a modest quantity of sodium happens normally in food sources. Most sodium is added during handling.
Try not to add salt. Use spices or flavors to add flavor to food.
Cook. Cooking allows you to control how much sodium is in the food.

5. Limit liquor
Restricting liquor to short of one beverage daily for ladies or two beverages every day for men can assist with bringing down pulse. Be that as it may, drinking an excessive amount of liquor can raise the pulse by a few. It can likewise decrease the viability of circulatory strain meds.

6. Stop smoking

Smoking increments circulatory strain. Halting smoking assists lower with blooding pressure. It can likewise diminish the gamble of coronary illness and work on generally speaking wellbeing, potentially prompting a more extended life.

7. Get a decent night's rest

Unfortunate rest quality — getting less than six hours of rest consistently for a long time — can add to hypertension. Various issues can disturb rest, including rest apnea, a propensity to fidget, and general restlessness (a sleeping disorder).

Inform your medical care supplier as to whether you frequently experience difficulty dozing. Finding and treating the reason can assist with further developing rest. Nonetheless, on the off chance that you don't have rest apnea or a tendency to fidget, follow these basic ways to get more soothing rest.

Adhere to a rest plan. Hit the hay and wake up simultaneously every day. Attempt to keep a similar timetable on weeknights and ends of the week.

Make a serene space. That implies keeping the resting space cool, calm, and dim. Accomplish something loosening up in the prior hour of sleep time. That could incorporate scrubbing down or doing unwinding works out. Stay away from splendid light, for example, from a television or PC screen.

Watch what you eat and drink. Try not to hit the hay eager or stuffed. Stay away from enormous dinners near sleep time. Limit or stay away from nicotine, caffeine, and liquor near sleep time, too.

Limit rests. For the people who view resting during the day as accommodating, restricting rest to 30 minutes sooner in the day could assist the evening with dozing.

8. Decrease pressure

Long haul (constant) close-to-home pressure might add to hypertension. More examination is required on the impacts of pressure decrease strategies to see if they can lessen pulse.

In any case, it can't damage to figure out what causes pressure, like work, family, funds, or sickness, and track down ways of lessening pressure. Attempt the accompanying:

Try not to attempt to do it excessively. Plan your day and spotlight your needs. Figure out how to say no. Permit sufficient opportunity to finish what should be finished.

Center around issues you have some control over and make arrangements to tackle them. For an issue at work, converse with a manager. For struggle with children or life partner, track down ways of settling it.

Keep away from pressure triggers. For instance, if heavy traffic causes pressure, travel at an alternate time or take public transportation. Stay away from individuals who cause pressure if conceivable.

Make time to unwind. Take time every day to sit discreetly and inhale profoundly. Set aside a few minutes for pleasant exercises or side interests, like going for a stroll, cooking, or chipping in. Practice appreciation. Offering thanks to others can assist with lessening pressure.

9. Screen your circulatory strain at home and get customary exams

Home observation can assist you with watching your pulse. It can make specific your meds and way of life changes are working.

Home pulse screens are accessible broadly and without a solution. Converse with a medical care supplier about home checking before you get everything rolling.

Ordinary encounters with a supplier are likewise key to controlling pulse. If your circulatory strain is very much controlled, ask your supplier how frequently you want to take a look at it. You could look at it just one time each day or now and again.

10. Get support

Strong loved ones mean quite a bit to great well-being. They might urge you to deal with yourself, drive you to the consideration supplier's office or begin an activity program with you to keep your pulse low.

www.ingramcontent.com/pod-product-compliance
Lightning Source LLC
LaVergne TN
LVHW050341160826
845677LV00014B/3724